Galveston Diet

Burn Fat, Tame Hormones, and Take Back Your Life

Dr. Miles J. Cooper

Disclaimer

The information provided in The Galveston Diet: Burn Fat, Tame Hormones, and Take Support Your Life is intended for educational and informational purposes only. It is not a substitute for professional medical advice, diagnosis, or treatment. Always consult with a qualified healthcare provider before starting any new diet, exercise program, or supplement regimen, especially if you have existing medical conditions, are pregnant, or are taking medications.

The author and publisher make no guarantees regarding the results readers may achieve from following the recommendations in this book. Individual results may vary, and the content is provided "as is," without warranties or representations. The reader takes full responsibility for their choices and outcomes.

This book does not aim to diagnose, treat, or cure medical conditions. Use the information provided responsibly, and always prioritize professional guidance for your unique health needs.

Table of contents

Introduction

The journey to health and vitality is emotionally personal, frequently filled with difficulties that vibe unconquerable. For some, the battle to oversee weight, balance hormones, and recapture energy can appear endless. The Galveston Diet offers a new, science-based approach to address these challenges by focusing on the main drivers of weight gain and hormonal imbalances. This presentation makes way for how this weighty strategy can engage you to play command over your health, rethink your relationship with food, and recover the dynamic life you merit.

Why the Galveston Diet is Unique

Traditional eating regimens frequently focus exclusively on calorie limitation, offering nonexclusive arrangements that neglect to address the mind-boggling exchange between hormones, inflammation, and weight gain. The Galveston Diet isn't simply one more eating routine — it's a lifestyle change custom-fitted to the extraordinary hormonal movements and metabolic necessities of women, especially during perimenopause and menopause.

Not at all like one-size-fits-all strategies, this program underlines anti-inflammatory eating, intermittent fasting, and supplementing thick food varieties to make a practical arrangement that works with your body, not against it. By focusing on the science behind hormonal health and inflammation, the Galveston Diet outfits you with the devices to consume fat all the more effectively, reestablish harmony with your hormones, and upgrade your general prosperity.

What separates this diet is its accentuation on strengthening. As opposed to directing unbending guidelines, it gives a system you can adjust to your lifestyle. This implies you can appreciate enduring outcomes without forfeiting the food varieties you love or feeling caught by prohibitive rules.

The Connections Between Hormones and Weight Management

For women, hormonal changes play a huge part in weight management, especially during perimenopause and menopause. Variances in estrogen, insulin, and cortisol levels can prompt expanded fat storage, diminished energy, and elevated inflammation. Traditional dieting approaches frequently neglect these hormonal elements, leaving women feeling disappointed and crushed when their endeavors don't yield results.

Inflammation, a quiet supporter of weight gain, is another basic component. Persistent inflammation disturbs metabolic cycles, making it harder to get thinner and simpler to acquire. The Galveston Diet resolves these issues by focusing on anti-inflammatory food sources and lifestyle procedures that normally diminish inflammation and advance hormonal amicability.

This diet additionally perceives the significance of metabolic flexibility, the storage of your body to switch between burning carbs and fats for energy. A hormonal awkward nature can prevent this flexibility, prompting weight gain and weakness. By integrating intermittent fasting and supplement-rich food varieties, the Galveston Diet reestablishes this fundamental metabolic capability, making way for feasible fat loss and expanded vitality.

How this Guide Can Assist You with Changing Your Life?
Setting out on the Galveston Diet is in excess of a choice to get thinner — it's a promise to change your health, energy, and in general personal satisfaction. This book fills in as your extensive aide, outfitting you with the information and useful devices to implement the Galveston diet effectively.

-You will become familiar with the science behind the eating routine and its focus standards, including:
-Understanding the role of inflammation in weight gain and how to battle it with designated dietary decisions.
-Bridling the power of intermittent fasting to adjust hormones and enhance fat copying.
-Picking nutrient-dense food sources that fuel your body and advance long-term health.

As well as making sense of the eating routine's central ideas, this guide gives noteworthy techniques to assist you with conquering normal difficulties, remaining roused, and fabricating reasonable habits. Whether you're getting ready for get-togethers, exploring occupied timetables, or confronting levels, you'll track down viable exhortation to keep you on target.

This journey isn't tied in with accomplishing flawlessness; it's about progress. As you dig further into the Galveston Diet, you'll find how little, steady changes can prompt significant, enduring changes. You'll acquire the certainty to play command over your health and move others to do likewise.

An Individual Invitation to Recover Your Life
The Galveston Diet is a challenge to rediscover the best version of yourself. It's about more than weight loss — it's tied in with subduing the hormonal disarray, diminishing inflammation, and recovering the vitality that permits you to take part in life's minutes completely.

Assuming you've battled with counts calories that vibe unreasonably or have been left asking why your endeavors aren't yielding outcomes, this program offers another way forward. It's upheld by science, intended for women like you, and established in an emotional comprehension of the difficulties that accompany hormonal changes.

As you turn the pages of this book, you'll not just figure out how to implement the Galveston Diet but in addition reveal the devices to build a better, more joyful, and more lively future. Now is the ideal time to play support command over your health, tame your hormones, and consume fat such that feels engaging, not overpowering.

This is your moment to embrace a lifestyle that praises sustenance, balance, and the delight of living great. Welcome to the Galveston Diet. We should get everything rolling.

Part 1: Understanding the Galveston Diet

CHAPTER 1: THE SCIENCE BEHIND THE GALVESTON DIET

Weight management and overall health are often misconstrued as straightforward conditions of calories in versus calories out. In any case, present-day science uncovers that the human body is undeniably more perplexing, especially for women exploring hormonal changes. The Galveston Diet reclassifies traditional slimming down by tending to the hidden elements of inflammation and hormonal irregular characteristics. This section digs into the logical rules that structure the underpinning of this pivotal way to deal with weight loss and health.

The Role of Inflammation in Weight Gain

Inflammation is a characteristic insusceptible reaction intended to safeguard the body from injury and contamination. At the point when intense, it fills in as an imperative mending system. Notwithstanding, ongoing, poor-quality inflammation is an alternate story — one that straightforwardly adds to weight gain and persistent sicknesses like diabetes, cardiovascular circumstances, and metabolic conditions.

Persistent inflammation disturbs hormonal flagging, hindering the body's storage to manage craving, energy storage, and digestion. For example, raised degrees of support of fiery markers like C-reactive protein (CRP) are connected to insulin obstruction, a condition that makes it hard for the body to really handle blood sugar. This obstruction frequently prompts expanded fat storage, especially around the mid-region.

The Galveston Diet battles constant inflammation through designated anti-inflammatory eating. By focusing on nutrient-dense food sources like omega-3 unsaturated fats, antioxidant, and phytonutrient-rich vegetables, this diet decreases fiery reactions and reestablishes metabolic balance.

How Hormones Impact Fat Storage and Energy

Hormones go about as substance couriers that direct virtually every cycle in the body, from appetite and energy use to stress and sleep. For women, hormones like estrogen, insulin, and cortisol play urgent parts in fat storage and energy balance.

Estrogen: During perimenopause and menopause, estrogen levels decline, prompting changes in fat conveyance. This hormonal shift frequently brings about expanded stomach fat, even without changes in diet or movement levels.

Insulin: Known as the body's blood sugar controller, insulin helps transport blood sugar into cells for energy. In any case, when insulin levels are reliably high because of unfortunate dietary decisions or stress, the body becomes impervious to its belongings. This condition, known as insulin opposition, adds to fat storage and weight gain.

Cortisol: Frequently called the stress hormone, cortisol impacts fat storage, especially in the stomach region. Persistent stress and high cortisol levels make weight loss essentially seriously tested.

The Galveston Diet straightforwardly addresses these hormonal elements by integrating rehearses like intermittent fasting, which further develops insulin sensitivity, and anti-inflammatory food sources, which alleviate the hormonal interruptions brought about by persistent inflammation.

The Unique Standards of the Galveston Diet

The Galveston Diet stands apart because it's anything but a one-size-fits-all arrangement. All things considered, it is custom-fitted to meet the one-of-a-kind metabolic and hormonal necessities of women, especially during midlife. Its three focus standards — anti-inflammatory eating, intermittent fasting, and nutrient-dense filling — make a synergistic impact that supports fat loss, hormonal balance, and general health.

1. Anti-inflammatory Eating: This rule includes devouring food sources that effectively lessen inflammation in the body. These include:

-Healthy fats like avocados, nuts, seeds, and greasy fish.

-Fiber-rich vegetables like spinach, kale, and broccoli.

Spices like turmeric and ginger, have anti-inflammatory properties.

By focusing on these food sources and limiting favorable to fiery things like refined sugars and handled food sources, the eating routine establishes an inward climate helpful for weight loss and recovery.

2. Intermittent fasting: Dissimilar to protocol calorie-cutting strategies, intermittent fasting stresses when you eat instead of the amount you eat. This training:

Further develops insulin sensitivity.

. Improves metabolic flexibility, permitting the body to switch between burning carbs and fats for energy.

. Upholds autophagy, a cell-fix process that lessens inflammation and lifts energy levels.

3. Nutrient-Dense Fueling: Each feast in the Galveston Diet is a chance to support the body. By focusing on great proteins, solid fats, and low-glycemic sugars, this approach guarantees you stay fulfilled while supporting ideal hormonal capability.

Interfacing Science to Supportable Outcomes

What compels the Galveston Diet manageable is its establishment in logical exploration and its versatility to individual lifestyles. For example, concentrates on showing that anti-inflammatories consume fewer calories advance weight loss as well, and diminish the gamble of constant ailments like joint pain, coronary illness, and diabetes. Essentially, research on intermittent fasting features its advantages for working on metabolic health and supporting long-term fat loss.

As opposed to pursuing transient outcomes, this diet focuses on enduring health and vitality. By tending to the underlying drivers of weight gain — hormonal irregular characteristics and ongoing inflammation — it engages you to accomplish your objectives without depending on prohibitive or unreasonable practices.

A New Approach to deal with Women's Health

The Galveston Diet is in excess of a weight loss plan; it's an upheaval by the way we get it and move toward women' health. It perceives that hormonal changes are not hindrances but rather amazing chances to advance health through science-supported techniques. By diminishing inflammation, adjusting hormones, and focusing on nutrient-dense food varieties, the eating routine establishes the groundwork for a better, more energetic you.

As you proceed with your journey through this book, you'll uncover noteworthy strategies to carry out these standards and change your way to deal with health and health. With the Galveston Diet, you're not simply counting calories — you're embracing a lifestyle intended to assist you with burning fat, tame hormones, and reclaim your life.

CHAPTER 2: HORMONES AND FAT LOSS

Hormones are the uncelebrated but truly great individuals of the body, coordinating essentially every interaction, from controlling craving and digestion to managing energy levels and state of mind. However, for some women, especially those coming from perimenopause and menopause, hormonal irregular characteristics become a significant snag to keeping a healthy weight. The Galveston Diet is extraordinarily intended to address these hormonal changes, giving a guide to recovering your health, vitality, and certainty.

Figuring Out Hormonal Imbalances: Estrogen, Insulin, And Cortisol
For most women, the journey to hormonal unevenness starts quietly but can grow into a fountain of side effects that influence weight, energy, and overall prosperity. Three essential hormones — estrogen, insulin, and cortisol — are especially significant in fat loss and weight management.

Estrogen:
Estrogen plays a critical part in managing muscle versus fat dissemination. Before menopause, women will generally store fat in the hips and thighs, an example connected to conceptive health. As estrogen levels decline during perimenopause and menopause, this fat conveyance shifts, with more fat gathering around the midsection. This "instinctive fat" isn't just difficult but additionally connected with expanded inflammation and uplifted dangers of cardiovascular sickness and diabetes.

Insulin:
Insulin is the hormone liable for shipping blood sugar from the circulatory system into cells for energy. Nonetheless, eating less high in refined carbs and sugars can prompt insulin obstruction — a state where the body battles to handle blood sugar. Insulin opposition triggers fat storage, especially in the stomach district, and makes weight loss testing despite dietary or exercise endeavors.

Cortisol:

Known as the stress hormone, cortisol influences how the body utilizes fats, proteins, and starches. Persistent stress can hoist cortisol levels, empowering the storage of fat, particularly around the abdomen. Furthermore, high cortisol levels frequently lead to expanded desires for sweet and greasy food sources, creating a pattern of weight gain and hormonal interruption.

The Galveston Diet recognizes the complicated interaction of these hormones and consolidates designated systems to rebalance them through diet and lifestyle changes.

The Effect of Perimenopause and Menopause On Weight

The progress into perimenopause and menopause is a characteristic phase of life, but it frequently accompanies unwanted changes, especially in weight and body organization. As estrogen levels drop, the metabolic rate diminishes, and the body turns out to be less effective at burning calories. Simultaneously, declining estrogen influences the development of leptin and ghrelin — hormones that control hunger and fullness — frequently prompting expanded craving and gorging.

Another key variable is the decrease in bulk, a condition known as sarcopenia, which further lessens metabolic productivity. Joined with hormonal vacillations, this makes a powerful coincidence for weight gain, especially as instinctive fat.

While these progressions are regular, they are not unconquerable. The Galveston Diet offers solutions tailored to the unique difficulties of midlife, focusing on anti-inflammatory food and intermittent fasting to battle these hormonal moves and support fat loss.

How the Galveston Diet Addresses Hormonal Difficulties?

The foundation of the Galveston Diet is its all-encompassing way to deal with adjusting hormones and supporting feasible fat loss. This is the way its key standards address hormonal difficulties:

1. Lessening Inflammation:

Persistent inflammation worsens hormonal irregular characteristics, making a pattern of weight gain and metabolic brokenness. The Galveston Diet's accentuation on anti-inflammatory food sources — like salad greens, greasy fish, and berries — mitigates these impacts, establishing a climate where hormones can work ideally.

2. Further developing Insulin Responsiveness:

Intermittent fasting, a focus part of the eating regimen, has been displayed to further develop insulin responsiveness. By expanding the periods between meals, the has the opportunity and energy to settle blood sugar levels and decrease insulin creation. This guides in fat loss as well as diminishes the gamble of creating type 2 diabetes.

3. Supporting Hormonal Balance:

The eating routine focuses on supplementing thick food sources plentiful in nutrients, minerals, and phytoestrogens — plant-based intensifies that copy the impacts of estrogen in the body. Food varieties like flaxseeds, soy, and lentils offer regular help for women encountering hormonal changes.

4. Promoting Stress Management:

Stress is a critical supporter of hormonal irregular characteristics. While diet is a pivotal part, the Galveston Diet likewise supports integral practices like care and ordinary activity to bring down cortisol levels and cultivate emotional prosperity.

The Science Behind These Strategies

Logical examination highlights the adequacy of tending to hormonal lopsided characteristics through diet and lifestyle. For instance:

-Studies have demonstrated the way that consumes less calories wealthy in anti-inflammatory food varieties can decrease markers of inflammation, like CRP, and further develop insulin responsiveness.

-Research on intermittent fasting features its advantages for hormonal health, including improved fat-copying limit and decreased insulin levels.

-A review distributed in The Diary of Endocrinology found that phytoestrogens in food sources like soy and flaxseeds might assist with reducing side effects of menopause, including weight gain.

By lining up with these evidence-based standards, the Galveston Diet gives a commonsense structure to women trying to deal with their weight and work on their health during midlife and then some.

Enabling Women to Play Control

Hormonal irregular characteristics and midlife weight gain can feel overpowering, however, the Galveston Diet is intended to enable women with the tools and information to regain control. By tending to the main drivers of fat stockpiling — as opposed to simply treating side effects — it offers a sustainable, science-supported way to deal with fat loss and general health.

Through deliberate decisions and informed systems, you can adjust your hormones, diminish inflammation, and accomplish a better, more energetic you. In the parts ahead, you'll investigate noteworthy stages to coordinate the Galveston Diet into your life and experience its groundbreaking advantages firsthand.

CHAPTER 3: CORE PRINCIPLES OF THE GALVESTON DIET

The Galveston Diet stands separated from traditional weight loss plans by focusing on the underlying drivers of weight gain as opposed to simply calorie counting. It is based on three extraordinary standards: anti-inflammatory eating, intermittent fasting, and filling your body with the right nutrients. These standards are intended to reestablish hormonal balance, decrease inflammation, and support maintainable fat loss while enabling you to feel invigorated and amazing.

Anti-inflammatory Eating

Inflammation is a characteristic interaction the body uses to mend wounds and battle diseases. In any case, persistent inflammation — frequently brought about by unfortunate dietary decisions, stress, and hormonal lopsided characteristics — can add to weight gain, weakness, and a large group of constant medical problems. The Galveston Diet tends to do this by focusing on food varieties that lessen inflammation and barring those that worsen it.

The Best Anti-inflammatory Food sources

Salad Greens: Spinach, kale, and arugula are plentiful in antioxidant like L-ascorbic acid and beta-carotene, which assist with combatting oxidative stress.

Greasy Fish: Salmon, mackerel, and sardines are high in omega-3 unsaturated fats, known to decrease inflammation and support heart health.

Berries: Blueberries, raspberries, and strawberries are loaded with anthocyanin's, intensifying that lessen inflammation and safeguard against cell harm.

Nuts and Seeds: Almonds, pecans, flaxseeds, and chia seeds give solid fats and fiber to settle blood sugar and diminish inflammation.

Spices: Turmeric, ginger, and cinnamon have anti-inflammatory properties and improve the kind of meal normally.

Food sources to Keep away from

Certain food sources are known to set off inflammation, disturb hormones, and prevent weight loss. These include:

. Processed foods high in trans fats and added substances.

. Refined sugars, like white bread and cakes.

. Sweet refreshments and snacks.

. Exorbitant alcohol utilization.

By making anti-inflammatory food sources the underpinning of your meals, you can establish a climate in your body that supports fat loss and hormonal health.

Intermittent fasting for Hormonal Health

Intermittent fasting (IF) is an incredible asset in the Galveston Diet, for calorie control as well as for its significant effect on hormones and digestion. In contrast to prohibitive weight control plans, IF focusses around when you eat as opposed to what you eat, giving your body the time it necessities to reset and fix.

How Intermittent Fasting Functions

During fasting periods, insulin levels drop, urging your body to consume and put away fat for energy. All the while, levels of human Growth hormone (HGH) increment, advancing fat consumption and muscle safeguarding. This hormonal shift lessens fat storage and empowers better digestion.

Benefits for Hormonal Health

Further developed Insulin Responsiveness: Fasting diminishes insulin obstruction, which is basic for preventing and managing weight gain, particularly in midlife.

Settled Cortisol Levels: An organized eating timetable can assist with managing cortisol, limiting stress related fat storage.

Upgraded Fat-burning: By broadening the time between meals, your body figures out how to depend on fat stores for energy, advancing sustainable weight loss.

Fasting Protocols That Fit Your Lifestyle
The Galveston Diet empowers flexibility in picking a fasting protocol that suits your everyday practice. Well-known choices include:

-16:8 Strategy: Fasting for 16 hours and eating during an 8-hour window.
-14:10 Strategy: A more available choice, fasting for 14 hours with a 10-hour eating window.
-24-Hour Quick: Performed on more than one occasion per week for cutting-edge specialists.

Fasting ought to be drawn nearer with care, particularly for women with exceptional hormonal requirements. Pay attention to your body, and make sure to fasting periods if essential.

Energizing Your Body with The Right Nutrients
The Galveston Diet stresses nutrient-dense food sources to help your body's energy needs, hormonal balance, and generally speaking health. Legitimate sustenance guarantees that your body has the instruments to work ideally, in any event, during fasting periods.

Focusing on Macronutrients
1. Solid Fats:
Tracked down in avocados, olive oil, and nuts, solid fats are a foundation of the Galveston Diet. They balance out blood sugar, lessen inflammation, and keep you feeling full and fulfilled.

2. Quality Proteins:
Lean meats, fish, eggs, and plant-based sources like tofu and lentils give fundamental amino acids to muscle fix, energy creation, and hormonal health.

3. Low-Glycemic Sugars:

Complex carbs like quinoa, yams, and vegetables give consistent energy without spiking insulin levels.

Micronutrient-Rich Food sources

Nutrients and minerals play a basic part in managing hormones and lessening inflammation. For instance:

. Vitamin D: Supports bone health and insusceptible capability. Tracked down in greasy fish and sustained food sources.

. Magnesium: Diminishes stress and further develops sleep quality. Tracked down in mixed greens, nuts, and seeds.

. Zinc: Advances hormone creation and resistant health. Tracked down in shellfish, beans, and entire grains.

Balancing Flexibility and Consistency

While the Galveston Diet gives clear rules, it likewise perceives the significance of flexibility. The objective isn't flawlessness however progress. Building meals around anti-inflammatory, nutrient-dense food sources and integrating fasting plans that work for you considers maintainable, long-term achievement.

Making a New Relationship with Food

By focusing in on these focus standards, the Galveston Diet encourages a better relationship with food. Rather than seeing meals as a wellspring of stress or culpability, you'll start to see them as any opportunities to feed your body and supporting your health.

The Galveston Diet isn't about hardship; it's about strengthening. By adjusting your dietary patterns with your body's normal rhythms and necessities, you can diminish inflammation, balance hormones, and accomplish enduring fat loss.

In the parts to come, you'll figure out how to implement these standards in pragmatic, noteworthy ways of changing your lifestyle and recover your health.

Part 2: Getting Started with the Galveston Diet

CHAPTER 4: PREPARING FOR SUCCESS

Leaving on the Galveston Diet is in excess of a dietary shift — it's a journey to change your relationship with food, hormones, and your general health. Readiness is fundamental to guarantee a smooth change into this lifestyle. By defining clear objectives, establishing a strong climate, and furnishing yourself with the right devices and assets, you establish the groundwork for long-term achievement.

Putting forth Reasonable Objectives and Assumptions
The way to progress on the Galveston Diet is to move toward it with clear, feasible objectives and reasonable assumptions. Weight loss, hormonal balance, and decreased inflammation take time and consistency, but the advantages go past the scale.

Define Your "Why"
Understanding the reason why you're chasing after the Galveston Diet gives inspiration and clearness. Is it true or not that you are looking for more energy, further developed hormone balance, or feasible fat loss? Record your reasons and return to them frequently to keep on track.

Make Brilliant Objectives
Put forth objectives that are Specific, Quantifiable, Attainable, Significant, and Time-bound:

. Specific: "I need to shed 10 pounds by decreasing inflammation and eating nutrient-dense food varieties."
. Quantifiable: Track progress through photographs, estimations, or diary sections.
. Reachable: Hold support nothing pounds of fat loss each week rather than ridiculous quick changes.
. Important: Adjust objectives to your more extensive health and health yearnings.

. Time-bound: Set a course of events for achievements to keep up with concentration and inspiration.

Focus around Non-Scale Triumphs

While weight loss may be one of your objectives, perceive different victories:

. Further developed energy levels.

. Better sleep quality.

. Less desires.

. More clear skin or diminished swelling.

These successes support your advancement and empower consistency.

Clearing Your Storage Room and Loading Up on Basics

Your current circumstance plays a basic part in molding your habits. Setting up your kitchen with anti-inflammatory food sources and eliminating triggers guarantees you're prepared for progress.

Lead a Storeroom Review

Eliminate food sources that advance inflammation or frustrate progress, for example,

-Sweet tidbits and drinks.

-Refined grains like white bread and pasta.

-Processed food sources high in trans fats or counterfeit added substances.

-Alcohol, particularly in overabundance.

You don't need to squander these things — give unopened, durable food sources to neighborhood good cause or food banks.

Stock Up on Galveston Diet Fundamentals

Fill your kitchen with nutrient-dense, anti-inflammatory food sources that line up with the eating routine's standards:

. Healthy Fats: Olive oil, avocado, nuts, seeds, and greasy fish.

. Lean Proteins: Chicken, turkey, eggs, and plant-based choices like lentils or tofu.

. Low-Glycemic Carbs: Yams, quinoa, and different non-bland vegetables.

. Flavor Enhancers: Spices, spices, and normal sugars like stevia or priest natural product.

Having these fixings promptly accessible limits the impulse to wander from the eating routine and guarantees meal readiness is consistent.

Arrange Your Kitchen

A coordinated kitchen diminishes stress and saves time:

-Arrange ingredients: Keep oils, spices, and grains in discrete areas.

-Utilize Clear Compartments: Store storage room staples in named, straightforward holders for simple access.

-Prep Produce: Wash and slice vegetables ahead of time to smooth out feast prep.

Tools and Assets to Help Your Journey

Having the right devices and assets can make taking on the Galveston Diet simpler and more agreeable.

Kitchen Tools

. Quality Cookware: Put resources into non-poisonous, sturdy pots and container.

. Blender or Food Processor: Ideal for making smoothies, sauces, or soups.

. Feast Prep Compartments: Utilize partitioned, reusable holders to store pre-arranged meals and snacks.

. Advanced Scale: For precisely estimating segments, particularly during the beginning phases.

Following Tools

-Diary or Application: Track meals, fasting windows, and progress. Applications like MyFitnessPal or Carb Chief can assist with checking supplement consumption.

-Wearables: Gadgets like Fitbit or Apple Watch track movement levels and sleep, giving bits of knowledge into what your lifestyle changes mean for your health.

Encouraging groups of people

. Online communities: Join bunches devoted to the Galveston Diet to share tips, recipes, and inspiration.

. Responsibility Accomplices: Band together with a companion or relative who can energize you during your journey.

. Proficient Direction: Consider counseling a nutritionist or dietitian acquainted with the Galveston Diet for customized guidance.

Building a Strong Mindset

Mindset is essentially as basic as readiness while changing to another lifestyle. Developing a positive, development situated point of view can make difficulties more reasonable and the journey seriously fulfilling.

Embrace Flexibility

The Galveston Diet isn't about flawlessness. Permit space for changes as you realize what turns out best for your body. Life will toss curves, however remaining focused on the general standards guarantees long-term achievement.

Observe Little Wins

Each forward-moving step merits praising, regardless of how little. Recognize achievements like finishing a fruitful fasting day or making a delectable anti-inflammatory meal.

Remain Patient and Constant

Change takes time. At the point when progress feels slow, advise yourself that enduring change requires consistency and versatility.

Associating Preparation to Progress

Planning for the Galveston Diet isn't just about clearing out your storeroom or purchasing the right instruments — it's tied in with getting yourself positioned for a sustainable, satisfying lifestyle. The time and effort you put resources into readiness will pay off as you explore the eating routine's focus standards and start to get brings about your energy levels, hormonal health, and overall prosperity.

By focusing on your objectives, coordinating your current circumstance, and outfitting yourself with the right tools, you'll be prepared to set out on this groundbreaking journey with certainty and clearness. In the following parts, you'll plunge further into the particulars of anti-inflammatory food varieties, meal plans, and fasting procedures that will assist you with flourishing.

CHAPTER 5: ANTI-INFLAMMATORY FOODS AND MEAL PLANS

The foundation of the Galveston Diet is its attention on anti-inflammatory eating. Constant inflammation is a quiet disruptor of health, adding to weight gain, hormonal imbalances, and a large group of ongoing diseases. By focusing on food sources that decrease inflammation and support your body, the Galveston Diet gives a pathway to further developed energy, better hormonal balance, and sustainable fat loss. This part investigates the best anti-inflammatory food sources, how to make adjusted meals, and gives an example 7-day meal plan to launch your journey.

The Best Food Sources for Lessening Inflammation

Anti-inflammatory food varieties work in cooperative energy with your body to bring down oxidative stress, manage hormones, and work on metabolic health. Integrating these food sources into your eating regimen guarantees you're energizing your body with the nutrients it requires to flourish.

-Healthy Fats: The Underpinning of Hormonal Health

Solid fats are fundamental for decreasing inflammation and supporting hormonal balance. They give enduring energy, settle blood sugar levels, and advance satiety.

-Olive Oil: Wealthy in monounsaturated fats and cell antioxidant, it's a staple of anti-inflammatory eating.

-Avocados: Loaded with solid fats, fiber, and nutrients like potassium.

-Nuts and Seeds: Almonds, pecans, flaxseeds, and chia seeds are incredible wellsprings of omega-3 unsaturated fats and other anti-inflammatory nutrients.

-Greasy Fish: Salmon, mackerel, and sardines give omega-3 unsaturated fats, which decrease fiery markers in the body.

-Energetic Vegetables: Nature's Supplement Powers to be reckoned with

-Vegetables are stacked with cancer prevention agents, nutrients, and minerals that battle inflammation and advance overall health.

-Mixed Greens: Spinach, kale, and Swiss chard are rich in cancer prevention agents like quercetin and kaempferol.

-Cruciferous Vegetables: Broccoli, cauliflower, and Brussels sprouts contain sulforaphane, a compound with strong anti-inflammatory properties.

-Beautiful Vegetables: Peppers, carrots, and beets add a variety of antioxidants and phytonutrients.

-Low-Glycemic Natural Products: Pleasantness Without the Spike

-Organic products with a low glycemic record give normal pleasantness and fundamental nutrients without causing blood sugar spikes.

-Berries: Blueberries, strawberries, and raspberries are high in anthocyanins, which battle inflammation.

-Citrus Organic products: Oranges, lemons, and grapefruits give L-ascorbic acid and flavonoids.

-Apples and Pears: These fiber-rich organic products support stomach health and manage processing.

Protein for Fix and Satiety

Protein plays a significant part in muscle fixing, metabolic health, and keeping you full between meals.

-Lean Animal Proteins: Chicken, turkey, and eggs are incredible wellsprings of excellent protein.

-Plant-Based Proteins: Lentils, beans, and tofu give protein along with fiber and fundamental nutrients.

-Herbs and Spices: Little Increments, Enormous Effect

Spices and spices add flavor to meals while conveying powerful anti-inflammatory compounds.

-Turmeric: Contains curcumin, a strong anti-inflammatory and antioxidant

-Ginger: Decreases inflammation and further develop processing.

-Garlic: Offers sulfur intensifies that help insusceptible and cardiovascular health.

-Entire Grains and Vegetables: Maintainable Energy Sources

Entire grains and vegetables give fiber, nutrients, and minerals while holding inflammation under wraps.

-Quinoa: A sans gluten grain loaded with protein and fiber.

-Oats: Contain beta-glucans, which diminish inflammation and further develop cholesterol levels.

-Beans and Lentils: High in fiber, protein, and cancer prevention agents.

Making Adjusted, Nutrient-dense Meals

Making meals that line up with the Galveston Diet's standards is both basic and fulfilling. Focus around balance, consolidating healthy fats, lean proteins, and low-glycemic sugars into every feast.

The Galveston Plate Strategy

Picture your plate isolated into segments:

. Half Vegetables: Fill around 50% of your plate with beautiful, non-boring vegetables.

. Quarter Protein: Add a serving of lean protein or plant-based other options.

. Quarter Healthy Fats and Grains: Incorporate a little part of solid fats and, alternatively, entire grains or vegetables.

Meal Planning Tips

. Clump Cooking: Plan huge parts of proteins, grains, and vegetables to blend and match over time.

. Pre-Part Snacks: Keep nuts, seeds, and cut vegetables prepared for fast, healthy eating.

. Use Flavor Wisely: Trial with spices, spices, and citrus to keep meals invigorating.

Test 7-DAY Meal PLAN

The accompanying meal plan gives an organized manual for integrating anti-inflammatory food varieties into your eating regimen. Every day incorporates nutrient-dense meals that are not difficult to plan and tasty.

Day 1

-Breakfast: Avocado toast on entire grain bread with a poached egg and spinach.

-Lunch: Barbecued chicken plate of mixed greens with blended greens, cherry tomatoes, pecans, and olive oil dressing.

-Supper: Prepared salmon with quinoa and simmered broccoli.

-Snack: Greek yogurt with blueberries and chia seeds.

Day 2

-Breakfast: Berry smoothie with almond milk, spinach, flaxseeds, and protein powder.

-Lunch: Lentil soup with a side of leafy greens and lemon dressing.

-Supper: Turkey meatballs with zucchini noodles and marinara sauce.

-Snack: Cut apple with almond spread.

Day 3

-Breakfast: Fried eggs with turmeric, sautéed kale, and avocado.

-Lunch: Quinoa salad with cooked vegetables, chickpeas, and tahini dressing.

-Supper: Barbecued shrimp with cauliflower rice and steamed asparagus.

-Snack: Hummus with carrot and cucumber sticks.

Day 4

-Breakfast: Greek yogurt parfait with granola, raspberries, and honey.

-Lunch: Barbecued chicken wrap with avocado, lettuce, and chime peppers in an entire grain tortilla.

-Supper: Dish singed cod with wild rice and sautéed spinach.

-Snack: Small bunch of blended nuts.

Day 5

-Breakfast: Chia pudding made with almond milk, finished off with cut banana and cinnamon.

-Lunch: Blended greens salad in with fish, olives, cucumber, and olive oil dressing.

-Supper: Sautéed tofu with bok choy, mushrooms, and earthy colored rice.

-Snack: Dull chocolate square with green tea.

Day 6

-Breakfast: Oats with almond spread, cut pears, and a sprinkle of flaxseeds.

-Lunch: Turkey and avocado lettuce wraps with a side of cherry tomatoes.

-Supper: Prepared chicken thighs with yams and broiled Brussels sprouts.

-Snack: Curds with pineapple pieces.

Day 7

-Breakfast: Veggie omelet with spinach, tomatoes, and mushrooms, presented with avocado cuts.

-Lunch: Lentil and quinoa bowl with cooked red peppers and tahini dressing.

-Supper: Barbecued salmon with squashed cauliflower and steamed green beans.

-Snack: Celery sticks with almond spread.

Connecting Your Plate to Your Objectives

Embracing anti-inflammatory eating isn't just about weight loss — it's tied in with powering your body for ideal health, subduing hormones, and living with vitality. This section outfits you with the information and tools to make meals that are both delightful and lined up with the standards of the Galveston Diet. As you practice these techniques, you'll see physical changes as well as feel more in line with your body's requirements.

CHAPTER 6: INTERMITTENT FASTING MADE SIMPLE

Advantages of Intermittent Fasting for Hormonal Health

Intermittent fasting (IF) has arisen as a groundbreaking practice for working on hormonal balance, especially for people exploring weight management challenges connected to hormone vacillations. This eating design, which switches support and forth between times of eating and fasting, goes past calorie limitation — it is an incredible asset for metabolic health and hormonal guidelines.

One of the essential advantages of IF is its ability to lessen insulin obstruction. Insulin, a hormone that manages blood sugar levels, can turn out to be less compelling because of ongoing indulging, high-sugar eats less, or hormonal changes during perimenopause and menopause. Intermittent fasting settles blood sugar levels, decreasing the gamble of insulin obstruction and working with fat loss, especially in difficult regions like the midsection.

Fasting additionally energizes metabolic exchange, where the body changes from involving blood sugar as its essential fuel to burning put-away fat. This switch upholds weight loss as well as advances cell fix processes, for example, autophagy, which eliminates harmed cells and diminishes inflammation. Lower inflammation levels further add to work on hormonal balance, as persistent inflammation frequently upsets hormones like cortisol and estrogen.

In addition, Intermittent fasting can improve the creation of development hormone, which supports fat consumption and muscle conservation. For women confronting declining estrogen levels, the development hormone turns out to be much more basic in keeping up with bone thickness and metabolic health. Ultimately, fasting periods give the stomach-related framework a sleep, supporting stomach health — a critical figure hormonal guideline.

Fasting Protocols That Work with Your Lifestyle

Picking a fasting protocol that lines up with your lifestyle and physical requirements is fundamental for long-term achievement. The following are probably the most famous and versatile IF strategies:

1. 16/8 Strategy: This includes fasting for 16 hours and eating inside an 8-hour window, for example, from early afternoon to 8 PM. It is great for fledglings and fits consistently into most day to day schedules.

2. 5:2 Eating routine: In this strategy, members eat typically for five days every week and confine calorie consumption (500-600 calories) for the excess two non-sequential days. This flexibility is especially appealing to those with occupied plans.

3. Eat-Stop-Eat: This includes a 24-hour quick a few times per week. While viable, it requires more discipline and probably won't suit everybody, particularly novices.

4. Substitute Day Fasting: This plan shifts support and forth between long periods of typical eating and long periods of calorie limitation. It is exceptionally viable but might be trying for people requesting physical or mental roles.

5. Time-Limited Eating: This variety focus on burning all meals inside a particular period, for example, 10 AM to 6 PM. It is brilliant for individuals who are inclined toward a less inflexible fasting plan.

While choosing a protocol, consider your plan for getting work done, family responsibilities, energy levels, and clinical history. The key is to begin slowly and pay attention to your body, changing the fasting window on a case-by-case basis.

Tips to Remain focused

Intermittent fasting can be testing at first, but with the right procedures, you can explore these difficulties successfully:

. Slide into It: Start with a more limited fasting window, like 12 hours, and step by step increment the term as your body adjusts.

. Remain Hydrated: Drinking a lot of water during fasting periods is significant. Unsweetened home grown teas, dark espresso, and imbued water can likewise assist with stifling appetite and keep you invigorated.

. Plan Your Meals: Guarantee that you're eating windows incorporate nutrient-dense, adjusted meals that give the important macronutrients (proteins, fats, and starches) and micronutrients (nutrients and minerals).

. Monitor Appetite Signs: Perceive the distinction between real craving and ongoing eating designs. Fasting assists you foster a more emotional association with your body's regular signs.

. Remain Occupied: Participate in useful exercises during fasting hours to occupy yourself from food cravings. Perusing, working out, or seeking leisure activities can keep your psyche off food.

. Be Adaptable: Life can be unusual, and adhering unbendingly to a fasting timetable may not be plausible all the time. Permit yourself the effortlessness to change and refocus without culpability.

. Keep tabs on Your Development: Journaling your fasting process, including how you feel physically and inwardly, can assist with recognizing examples and regions for development.

Tending to Normal Concerns and Confusions

A few concerns and misinterpretations about intermittent fasting can deter individuals from attempting it. The following are a couple explained:

. Apprehension about Losing Muscle: that's what exploration shows IF, when joined with satisfactory protein admission and strength preparing, assists safeguard with muscling mass.

. Women and Fasting: While at the same time fasting can be advantageous for women, fitting the way to deal with hormonal needs is fundamental. Women ought to stay away from excessively prohibitive fasting designs that might upset periods or worsen hormonal lopsided characteristics.

. Hunger During Fasting: Yearning will in general diminish over the long-term as the body adjusts to putting away fat for energy. Burning nutrient-dense meals during eating windows likewise makes a difference.

. Energy Levels: Many individuals report expanded mental lucidity and stable energy levels after adjusting to intermittent fasting, as opposed to the conviction that fasting prompts exhaustion.

Intermittent fasting and Long-term Health

The advantages of intermittent fasting stretch out past weight loss. Studies show its role in decreasing the gamble of ongoing sicknesses like sort 2 diabetes, cardiovascular illness, and Alzheimer's. Furthermore, the accentuation on careful eating and organized feast times can encourage a better relationship with food.

By coordinating intermittent fasting into your lifestyle, you can encounter worked on hormonal health, reasonable weight management, and upgraded general prosperity. With tolerance, constancy, and a customized approach, intermittent fasting can turn into a useful asset in your health process.

Part 3: Strategies to Burn Fat and Tame Hormones

CHAPTER 7: THE ROLE OF EXERCISE IN THE GALVESTON DIET

Types of Exercises that Supplement the Eating Diet

Exercise plays an urgent part in upgrading the advantages of the Galveston Diet by advancing fat loss, supporting hormonal health, and working on general prosperity. To improve your outcomes, it's fundamental to pick exercise types that line up with the standards of the eating regimen and your wellness level.

1. Strength Training:

Strength training is one of the best activities for women, particularly during and after menopause. Building bulk helps support digestion and checks the regular loss of muscle that happens with age. Strength training likewise upholds bone health, which can be undermined by hormonal changes. Consolidate exercises like squats, thrusts, deadlifts, and push-ups, or use obstruction groups and loads for a full-body exercise.

2. High-Intensity Interval Training (HIIT):

HIIT exercises shift support and forth between short eruptions of extreme movement and recovery periods, making them proficient in burning fat and working on cardiovascular health. This sort of activity increases insulin sensitivity and advances metabolic exchange, permitting your body to consume and put away fat productively. A 20-30-minute HIIT meeting, a few times each week, can yield huge advantages.

3. Low-Effect Cardio:

For the individuals who favor gentler types of activity, strolling, swimming, or cycling are incredible choices. These exercises support heart health, decrease stress, and supplement the anti-inflammatory standards of the Galveston Diet.

4. Yoga and Pilates:

These activities are especially valuable for stress management and flexibility. Yoga and Pilates further develop stance, balance, and focus strength, which are all fundamental for overall prosperity. They likewise improve care, assisting you with remaining associated with your body's requirements.

5. Functional Training:

Functional training focuses on developments that mirror ordinary exercises, further developing coordination and strength for everyday undertakings. These activities lessen the gamble of injury and supporting joint health.

Building a Maintainable Fitness Routine

Making a steady and pleasant workout routine is critical to keeping up with the physical and hormonal advantages of the Galveston Diet. This is the way to build a feasible arrangement:

Begin Little and Progress Continuously:

On the off chance that you're new to working out, start with short meetings, like 10-15 minutes every day, and continuously increment the length and power. Consistency is a higher priority than flawlessness.

Consolidate Different Exercise Types:

A reasonable schedule that incorporates strength training, cardio, and flexibility practices guarantees far-reaching benefits. Hold support nothing 150 minutes of moderate-power movement or 75 minutes of overwhelming action each week, as suggested by health rules.

Pay attention to Your Body:

Hormonal vacillations can influence energy levels, so it's critical to appropriately adjust your daily practice. On low-energy days, pick delicate exercises like extending or strolling rather than serious exercises.

Plan Your Exercises:

Deal with practice like some other significant responsibility by saving specific times in your schedule. Morning exercises can support energy and set an uplifting vibe for the afternoon, while night meetings can assist with easing stress.

Make It Charming:

Pick exercises you truly appreciate to guarantee long-term adherence. Moving, climbing, or group classes can change it up and be amusing to your everyday practice.

THE Significance of Sleep and Recovery

Sleep and recovery are in many cases neglected parts of a fitness routine however are basic for accomplishing enduring outcomes. Overtraining can increase cortisol levels, disturb sleep, and frustrate muscle fixes — checking the advantages of your exercises.

1. Integrate Sleep Days:

Plan somewhere around one to two sleep days of the week to permit your body to recuperate. Sleep doesn't mean latency; light exercises like yoga or strolling can in any case be incorporated.

2. Focus on Sleep:

Sleep is fundamental for muscle recovery and hormonal guidelines. Go for the gold long stretches of value sleep each evening. Make a sleep schedule that incorporates unwinding methods, like perusing or contemplation, to help better sleep.

3. Practice Active Recovery:

On recovery days, take part in low-power exercises like stretching, froth rolling, or comfortable strolls. These exercises elevate the blood stream to muscles and assist with diminishing inflammation.

4. Hydrate and Refuel:

Proper hydration and sustenance are vital for recovery. After exercises, consume a meal or bite that incorporates protein and starches to renew energy stores and support muscle fix.

Exercise and Hormonal Balance

Exercise significantly affects hormonal health, making it a fundamental part of the Galveston Diet. This is the way standard physical work impacts key hormones:

. Insulin: Exercise improves insulin responsiveness, assisting the body with utilizing blood sugar all the more really and lessening the gamble of insulin opposition.

. Cortisol: Moderate-power exercise can bring down cortisol levels, relieving the effect of persistent weight on weight and general health.

. Estrogen and Progesterone: Strength training and cardio can assist with adjusting these hormones, which play a significant part in digestion, state of mind, and energy levels.

. Growth Hormone: Exercise invigorates the creation of development hormone, which supports fat consumption, muscle development, and tissue fix.

. Endorphins: physical activity discharges endorphins, further developing mindset and lessening stress, which is particularly significant during hormonal advances like menopause.

Conquering Exercise Difficulties

While the advantages of exercise are irrefutable, confronting obstacles is normal. This is the way to address them:

. Absence of Time: Consolidate more limited exercises, similar to 10-minute strength or HIIT meetings, and focus on exercises that convey the greatest advantages in negligible time.

. Low Energy Levels: Change your daily practice to incorporate gentler activities, and guarantee you're powering your body with nutrient-dense food sources.

. Inspiration Downturns: Set specific, feasible objectives and celebrate little triumphs. Banding together with an exercise mate or joining a wellness gathering can likewise support responsibility and excitement.

. Physical Limitations: Counsel a medical care supplier or wellness expert to plan a modified schedule that obliges any wounds or constraints.

The Drawn-out Advantages of a Functioning Lifestyle
Integrating regular exercise into your Galveston Diet venture offers help that extends past fat loss. Improved cardiovascular health, upgraded versatility, more grounded bones, and a more prominent feeling of prosperity are only a couple of the prizes. By embracing a reasonable and maintainable way to deal with fitness, you're supporting your ongoing health objectives as well as putting resources into a vibrant and active future.

With the right attitude, assets, and devotion, exercise can turn into a vital and charming piece of your lifestyle, supplementing the groundbreaking power of the Galveston Diet.

CHAPTER 8: MANAGING STRESS AND SLEEP FOR HORMONAL BALANCE

The Stress-Weight Connection

Stress is in excess of an emotional encounter; it's a physiological reaction with critical ramifications for your hormonal health and weight management. At the point when you experience stress, your body initiates the "survival" reaction, delivering cortisol, a hormone intended to assist you with answering dangers. While useful in short explodes, constant stress can prompt tenaciously high cortisol levels, upsetting hormonal balance and adding to weight gain.

Cortisol impacts where and how your body stores fat, frequently prompting an expansion in instinctive fat around the mid-region. This kind of fat is connected to higher dangers of metabolic circumstances, including insulin obstruction and inflammation. Ongoing stress can likewise prompt indulging, especially desires for high-sugar and high-fat food varieties, as your body looks for fast energy to adapt to the apparent danger.

The Galveston Diet emphasizes managing stress to help hormonal balance and lessen inflammation. By tending to the main drivers of stress and carrying out viable ways of dealing with especially difficult times, you can limit its effect on your weight and generally speaking health.

Basic Stress Decrease Methods

Managing stress doesn't need a total lifestyle update. All things being equal, consolidating little, reliable practices into your everyday schedule can make a significant difference.

1. Care Practices:

Strategies like reflection, emotional breathing, and moderate muscle unwinding can assist with bringing down cortisol levels and work on your storage to adapt to stress. For example, saving 5-10 minutes every day for careful breathing can make a quieting schedule that grounds you during testing times.

2. Physical Activity:

Exercise is a characteristic stress reliever. Exercises like strolling, yoga, or swimming help your physical health as well as diminish stress by delivering endorphins, the body's vibe great hormones.

3. Journaling:

Recording your considerations and sentiments can assist you with handling feelings and distinguishing stress triggers. Appreciation journaling, specifically, has been displayed to work on mental prosperity by moving concentration toward positive encounters.

4. Using time productively:

Stress frequently originates from feeling overpowered. Focus on undertakings, delegate whenever the situation allows, and make a day to day plan that incorporates breaks for taking care of oneself.

5. Social Help:

Associating with loved ones can assist you with exploring stress all the more physically. Sharing your encounters and looking for help encourages emotional versatility.

Improving Sleep for Fat Loss and Energy

Sleep is a foundation of hormonal health and plays a basic part in weight management. During sleep, your body fixes and recovers tissues controls hormones, and cycles recollections. Unfortunate sleep disturbs these cycles, prompting irregular characteristics that can influence hunger, energy levels, and fat stockpiling.

Key hormones impacted by sleep include:

Leptin and Ghrelin: These hormones manage yearning and satiety. Lacking sleep diminishes leptin (the hormone that signals completion) and increments ghrelin (the hormone that triggers hunger), prompting gorging.

Insulin: Unfortunate sleep decreases insulin responsiveness, making it harder for your body to control blood sugar and store energy really.

Cortisol: Lack of sleep raises cortisol levels, further adding to stress and fat stockpiling.

Establishing A Climate that welcomes sleeps

To guarantee helpful sleep, fundamental to develop a climate upholds unwinding and limits interruptions.

1. Lay out a Sleep Timetable:

Hit the hay and wake up simultaneously every day, even on ends of the week. Consistency directs your body's inner clock, making it more straightforward to nod off and awaken feeling invigorated.

2. Limit Screen Time Before Bed:

The blue light discharged by telephones, tablets, and PCs obstructs melatonin creation, a hormone fundamental for sleep. Intend to switch off monitors essentially an hour prior to sleep time.

3. Make a Loosening up Sleep time Schedule:

Participate in quieting exercises, like perusing, cleaning up, or rehearsing delicate stretches, to indicate to your body that now is the ideal time to slow down.

4. Advance Your Sleep Environment:

Keep your room cool, dull, and calm. Consider utilizing power outage shades, a support ground noise, or a fan to improve solace. Put resources into an agreeable bedding and cushions to help relaxing sleep.

5. Limit Caffeine and Alcohol:

The two substances can slow down sleep quality. Try not to polish off caffeine in the early evening and cutoff alcohol admission, as it can upset emotional sleep cycles.

The Interaction Among Stress and Sleep

Stress and sleep are complicatedly associated, frequently impacting each other in a cycle. Ongoing stress can make it hard to fall or stay unconscious, while unfortunate sleep fuels feelings of anxiety and disables your storage to adapt to difficulties. Tending to both at the same time is basic for accomplishing hormonal balance and improving your health.

Strategies to Adjust Stress and Sleep Management

-Practice Evening Relaxation: Integrate care or delicate yoga into your sleep time routine to slip the change into sleep.

-Limit Energizers: Stay away from weighty meals, serious activity, or invigorating discussions near sleep time.

-Focus on Breath work: Procedures like the 4-7-8 breathing strategy can quiet your sensory system and set up your body for sleep.

Keeping tabs on Your Development

Observing your stress and sleep examples can give significant experiences into what your lifestyle changes are meaning for your health. Utilize a diary or a wearable gadget to follow the accompanying:

-Feelings of anxiety: Record stress triggers and survival techniques to recognize examples and regions for development.

-Sleep Quality: Note the span and nature of your sleep, including any disturbances, to recognize factors influencing tranquility.

Embracing the Long-term Advantages

By managing stress and focusing on sleep, you're not just supporting the standards of the Galveston Diet but in addition working on your general personal satisfaction. Decreased inflammation, better hormonal balance, and upgraded energy are only a couple of the prizes you'll insight.

Coordinating these practices into your everyday schedule can make a positive criticism circle, where adjusted hormones work on your storage to oversee stress and accomplish helpful sleep. Over the long-term, these progressions will support your obligation to the Galveston Diet and assist you with accomplishing enduring health and vitality.

CHAPTER 9: NUTRIENTS AND SUPPORTIVE STRATEGIES

Key Nutrients for Hormonal and Inflammatory Balance

Supplements can play a huge part in upgrading the impacts of the Galveston Diet by tending to nourishing holes, supporting hormonal balance, and decreasing inflammation. While food stays the establishment, designated supplementation gives an extra layer of help for ideal health. The following are key supplements to consider:

1. Omega-3 Unsaturated fats

Omega-3s are known for their strong anti-inflammatory properties. They assist with decreasing foundational inflammation, support cerebrum health, and advance heart health. Greasy fish like salmon and mackerel are great sources, but on the off chance that you don't consume these routinely, a top notch fish oil or green growth based omega-3 enhancement can fill the hole. Search for nutrients containing EPA (eicosapentaenoic acid) and DHA (docosahexaenoic corrosive) for greatest advantage.

2. Vitamin D

Fundamental for bone health, resistant capability, and hormonal guideline, vitamin D is much of the time lacking in numerous people. Satisfactory levels of this nutrient can further develop insulin responsiveness and lessen inflammation. A day to day supplement might be important, particularly for those with limited sun exposure. A straightforward blood test can decide your ongoing levels and guide fitting dosing.

3. Magnesium

Magnesium upholds north of 300 enzymatic cycles in the body, including hormone guideline, stress decrease, and further developed sleep quality. It can likewise ease side effects of perimenopause and menopause, for example, muscle issues and emotional episodes. Magnesium glycinate or citrate are emotionally bioavailable structures for supplementation.

4. Probiotics

Stomach health is essential to overall health and hormonal balance. A great probiotic supplement can further develop processing, lessen swelling, and supporting the stomach microbiome, which plays a part in directing inflammation and digestion.

5. Curcumin

The dynamic compound in turmeric, curcumin is eminent for its anti-inflammatory and cancer prevention agent properties. It can assist with lessening joint agony, battle inflammation, and supporting in general health. Matching curcumin with dark pepper upgrades its bioavailability.

6. B Vitamins

The B-complex nutrients, especially B6, B12, and folate, are fundamental for energy creation, synapse combination, and lessening inflammation. They likewise play a basic part in managing stress and supporting hormonal health.

When and how to Utilize Supplements Securely

Nutrients are best when utilized mindfully and related to a decent eating routine. Here are a few rules for protected and viable use:

. Talk with a Medical Services Supplier: Prior to beginning any enhancement routine, counsel a medical care proficient to guarantee similarity with your health status, meds, and dietary necessities.

. Quality Matters: Pick nutrients from legitimate brands that go through outsider testing for immaculateness and power. Search for certificates, for example, NSF or USP to guarantee great items.

. Begin with Low Portions: Start with the suggested least portion and monitor your body's reaction prior to expanding measurements.

. Be Consistent: Integrate nutrients into your day to day daily schedule simultaneously every day to lay out a propensity and boost benefits.

. Stay away from Over-Supplementation: More isn't better all the time. Unnecessary supplementation can prompt imbalances or aftereffects. For instance, high portions of vitamin D without observing can cause harmfulness.

Extra Treatments to Improve Results

Beyond supplements, a few steady treatments line up with the standards of the Galveston Diet and can additionally improve your journey toward hormonal balance and weight management.

1. Massage Therapy

Standard support massages decrease stress hormones like cortisol while expanding serotonin and dopamine, further developing temperament and unwinding. Massage likewise improves flow and lymphatic waste, helping with detoxification and decreasing inflammation.

2. Needle therapy

Established in traditional Chinese medication, needle therapy has been displayed to adjust hormones, reduce stress, and further develop sleep quality. It might likewise uphold weight management by checking craving and upgrading digestion.

3. Yoga and Brain Body Practices

Rehearses like yoga, jujitsu, and qigong join physical development with care, assisting with lessening stress, further develop flexibility, and supporting hormonal health. Ordinary practice can cultivate a more emotional association between your brain and body, supporting healthy habits.

4. Infrared Sauna Treatment

Infrared saunas advance detoxification through perspiring and may lessen inflammation and further develop flow. This treatment can supplement the anti-inflammatory focal point of the Galveston Diet.

5. Cognitive Behavioral Therapy (CBT)

For those battling with close to home eating or stress-related ways of behaving, CBT gives instruments to reexamine negative idea designs and foster better survival strategies.

Incorporating Strong Strategies into Your Lifestyle

Integrating supplements and treatments into your routine doesn't need to feel overpowering. This is the way to make it reasonable:

-Lay out a Daily schedule: Make an everyday timetable that incorporates supplement admission, exercise, and taking care of oneself practices like yoga or reflection.

-Keep tabs on Your Development: Utilize a diary or application to monitor changes in your energy levels, sleep quality, and overall health. This assists you with recognizing what's working and where changes are required.

-Remain Adaptable: Life occurs, and there might be days when you can't adhere to each part of your arrangement. Focus around consistency over flawlessness.

The Long-Term Advantages of Supplementation and Strong Treatments

By nicely incorporating nutrients and strong techniques, you can address the underlying drivers of hormonal irregular characteristics and inflammation. This comprehensive strategy intensifies the advantages of the Galveston Diet, prompting further developed energy, better weight management, and upgraded generally speaking health.

Keep in mind, supplements and treatments are devices to supplement — not supplant — a solid eating regimen and lifestyle. When utilized in a calculated manner, they can assist you with opening your body's true storage and keep up with hormonal concordance for quite a long time into the future.

Part 4: Living the Galveston Diet Lifestyle

CHAPTER 10: OVERCOMING COMMON CHALLENGES

Navigating Social Events and Dining Out

Keeping up with the Galveston Diet while mingling or feasting out can feel threatening, but it's far from impossible with readiness and careful decisions. Social environments frequently include rich food varieties, enticing treats, and friend stress that could challenge your responsibility. Notwithstanding, you can remain focused without feeling denied or separated.

Begin by preparing. On the off chance that you're going to a social event, propose to carry a dish lined up with the Galveston Diet standards. This guarantees there's somewhere around one choice that upholds your objectives while acquainting others with anti-inflammatory, nutrient-dense food sources. While feasting out, see the eatery's menu on the web and recognize meals that can be altered to suit your requirements. Settle on lean proteins, a lot of vegetables, and healthy fats like olive oil or avocado.

Powerful communication likewise plays a key part. Amiably however confidently share your dietary inclinations with companions or servers, stressing your emphasis on sustaining food varieties as opposed to limiting yourself. Whenever confronted with strain to enjoy, help yourself to remember your objectives and how far you've come.

At long last, practice balance and flexibility. It's alright to appreciate infrequent treats or adjust your strategy for extraordinary events. Focus around the general example of your eating regimen instead of confined occasions, and recall that one meal won't crash your advancement.

Remaining Consistent During Busy or Stressful Time

Life's requests can frequently disturb even the best-laid plans. Stress, rushed plans, and unforeseen difficulties can make it enticing to return to old habits. To beat these obstructions, readiness and mindset are urgent.

To begin with, focus on meal arranging and arrangement. Devote a particular time every week to design meals, staple shop, and get ready food. Clump cooking anti-inflammatory staples like simmered vegetables, barbecued proteins, and supplement stuffed soups can save time and guarantee you generally have healthy choices close by.

Time-impeding your timetable for meals, exercise, and taking care of oneself can assist with keeping up with consistency. Treat these exercises as non-debatable meetings with yourself. On the off chance that you're in a hurry, focus around little, significant activities — like a fast, nutrient-dense breakfast smoothie or a 10-minute walk.

Mindset matters as well. Rethink occupied periods as any opportunities to reaffirm your obligation to health. Instead of review difficulties as mishaps, consider them to be opportunities to build strength. Perceive that taking care of oneself is fundamental, particularly when life feels overpowering.

Finally, lean on your emotionally supportive network. Share your objectives with believed friends or relatives who can empower and persuade you. Joining an internet based local area zeroed in on the Galveston Diet can likewise give important assets and motivation.

Taking care of Plateaus and Adjusting Your Plan

Weight loss plateaus are a characteristic piece of any health venture. While they can be disappointing, they additionally signal a potential chance to rethink and calibrate your strategy. Understanding the purposes for plateaus and creating vital changes can assist you with conquering them.

Plateaus frequently happen on the grounds that your body adjusts to new habits over the long run, prompting a decreased calorie shortfall or more slow metabolic rate. To address this, begin by auditing your habits. Is it safe to say that you are inadvertently burning more calories or moving less? Saving a food and action diary for a couple of days can give lucidity.

Think about fluctuating your daily practice. Changing your intermittent fasting plan, integrating new anti-inflammatory food sources, or changing your activity routine can reconnect your digestion. For instance, in the event that you've been following a 16:8 fasting protocol, take a stab at broadening your fasting window somewhat or exploring different avenues regarding another day fasting approach.

Stress and sleep can likewise affect progress. Raised cortisol levels from constant stress or inadequate sleep can thwart fat loss. Focus on unwinding procedures and go for the gold long stretches of value sleep every evening.

At last, focus around non-scale victories. Recall that the Galveston Diet isn't exclusively about weight loss; it's about generally speaking health and hormonal balance. Supplements in energy, mind-set, and inflammation levels are similarly essentially as critical as changes on the scale.

Embracing Flexibility and Long-term Achievement
The Galveston Diet isn't about unbending principles or flawlessness — it's a sustainable lifestyle based on flexibility. Difficulties will emerge, but the way in which you answer them decides your drawn out progress.

Flexibility is critical. On the off chance that you go astray, fight the temptation to harp on difficulties. All things considered, pull together and return to your habits with a renewed feeling of direction. Consistency over the long-term matters undeniably more than intermittent slips up.

Commend your advancement, regardless of how little. Recognize achievements like getting ready meals reliably, finishing a fasting period, or pursuing better decisions during a bustling week. These accomplishments support your responsibility and keep you spurred.

Recollect that the Galveston Diet is a journey, not an objective. Each challenge you beat builds the abilities and certainty expected to support this lifestyle into the indefinite future. By remaining patient, industrious, and proactive, you can explore obstructions with effortlessness and keep on receiving the extraordinary rewards of this strategy.

CHAPTER 11: BUILDING LONG-TERM HABITS

Making the Galveston Diet a Sustainable Lifestyle

A definitive objective of the Galveston Diet isn't simply brief fat loss or hormonal balance but making a sustainable lifestyle that cultivates health and vitality. Building long-term habits requires a shift from transient fixes to well established, predictable practices that fit consistently into your everyday daily schedule.

A vital technique for maintainability is developing a mindset of progress over flawlessness. Life is brimming with changes — travel, festivities, and unexpected conditions — however these don't need to crash your endeavors. Rather than focusing in on faultless adherence, focus on consistency and flexibility. For instance, on the off chance that you can't follow your standard intermittent fasting plan, conform to a more limited fasting window. In the event that anti-inflammatory food sources aren't promptly accessible, go for the gold potential decisions and refocus at the following an open door.

Another primary part of long-term achievement is happiness. The Galveston Diet ought to feel fulfilling and invigorating as opposed to prohibitive. Investigate recipes that line up with the eating regimen's standards however invigorate your taste buds. Try different things with spices, spices, and various cooking styles to make meals agreeable and changed. At the point when you love what you eat, remaining predictable turns out to be natural.

Incorporate the eating regimen into your lifestyle by adjusting it to your qualities and needs. Assuming family meals are significant, include your friends and family in meal arranging and readiness. On the off chance that you esteem care, use meal times as an amazing chance to dial support and enjoy each snack. This arrangement assists the Galveston with counting calories feel like an expansion of who you are instead of a different, unbending arrangement.

Observing Progress without Flawlessness

Praising your progress is indispensable for inspiration and long-term adherence. In any case, the focus ought to extend beyond the scale. While weight loss is many times an objective, different triumphs — like superior energy, better sleep, or diminished inflammation — are similarly significant.

Track your successes through techniques that impact you. A diary can help catch non-scale triumphs, for example, lower feelings of anxiety, better processing, or expanded endurance during exercises. Commend these achievements with non-food rewards like a loosening up spa day, another exercise outfit, or quality time with friends and family.

It's likewise fundamental to perceive that difficulties are a characteristic piece of any journey. Rather than review them as disappointments, rethink them as learning amazing opportunities. For instance, if an end-of-the-week trip prompts decisions that don't line up with your objectives, ponder what could have assisted you with remaining focused and apply those examples later on.

Progress isn't straight, and that is completely fine. The objective is a consistent improvement over the long run, not short-term change. Embrace the little wins, remain patient with yourself, and recollect that each step in the right direction counts, regardless of how little.

Rousing Others to Join Your Journey

One of the most compensating parts of embracing the Galveston Diet is the valuable chance to motivate and uphold others in seeking their health objectives. At the point when friends, family, or associates see your change, they might be interested in your strategy and anxious to find out more.

Begin by sharing your experience legitimately. Discuss how the Galveston Diet has worked on your energy, mindset, or general health. Share your #1 recipes or viable tips for feast arranging and intermittent fasting. Keep the discussion positive, focusing on the advantages as opposed to outlining it as prohibitive or troublesome.

Show others how it's done. Your consistency and excitement can rouse others to move toward better habits. Whether it's intriguing a companion to go along with you for a meal prep meeting or empowering a colleague to attempt an intermittent fasting plan, little activities can make a far reaching influence.

It is likewise significant to Build a strong community. Think about joining or making a gathering — whether on the online or face to face — where individuals can share recipes, celebrate achievements, and empower each other. Having an organization of similar people encourages responsibility and brotherhood, making the journey more charming.

Keep in mind, that your process can rouse others without judgment or tension. Everybody's way to health is unique, and your role is to offer support and offer bits of knowledge that can assist them with finding what turns out best for them.

Focusing on A Long period OF Health

The Galveston Diet isn't simply a program — it's a pledge to deep-rooted health. By focusing on manageable habits, commending your accomplishments, and building a strong organization, you make an establishment for getting through health.

Health is dynamic, and your requirements might change after some time. Occasionally rethink your objectives, habits, and schedules to guarantee they line up with your ongoing lifestyle and needs. Remain open to learning and adjusting as new difficulties and potential opportunities emerge.

Eventually, the Galveston Diet is about strengthening. It equips you with the information and instruments to play control over your health, explore difficulties, and flourish. With commitment, flexibility, and an emphasis on long-term habits, you can support the extraordinary advantages of this strategy into the indefinite future, recovering your vitality and making every moment count.

Conclusion

The Galveston Diet is more than a plan for burning fat and adjusting hormones; it's an extraordinary way to deal with recovering your health and vitality. By understanding the effect of inflammation and hormonal imbalances on weight and prosperity, this guide enables you to settle on informed decisions custom fitted to your extraordinary requirements.

Through anti-inflammatory eating, intermittent fasting, and nutrient-dense meals, the Galveston Diet offers a reasonable way to fat loss and energy reclamation. It emphasizes the significance of comprehensive health, consolidating stress management, quality sleep, and customized fitness schedules for enduring outcomes. By celebrating progress, conquering difficulties, and building strong habits, you can make a lifestyle that encourages long-term achievement.

Right now is an ideal opportunity to make a move. Start with little, consistent moves — attempt another recipe, take on a fasting protocol, or clear your storage space of fiery food sources. Keep in mind, flawlessness isn't the objective; progress is.

The Galveston Diet is your guide to a better, more lively life. Embrace this journey with certainty, realizing you have the tools and information to succeed. Play responsibility for your health today, and move others to do likewise. The best version of yourself is reachable — go claim it.